a morning cup of
pilates ™

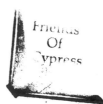

Published by Crane Hill Publishers
www.cranehill.com

Printed in Canada

Library of Congress Cataloging-in-Publication Data

Dorman, Marsha.
  A morning cup of pilates : one 15-minute routine to invigorate the body, mind, and spirit / Marsha K. Dorman.
     p. cm.
  ISBN 1-57587-221-8 (alk. paper)
  1. Pilates method. 2. Exercise. 3. Physical fitness. I. Title.
  RA781.D575 2004
  613.7'1--dc22
                                    2004004026

10   9   8   7   6   5   4   3   2   1

a morning cup of pilates ™

one 15-minute routine to invigorate
the body, mind, & spirit

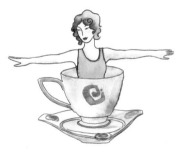

marsha k. dorman, m.s.p.t.

CRANE HILL
PUBLISHERS

Acknowledgments

I am grateful to the many gifted Pilates instructors who have inspired me, particularly Amy Taylor Alpers and Rachel Taylor Segel, owners of The Pilates Center—Boulder, whose teaching staff skillfully guided me on a journey of self-discovery that brought me face to face with myself and encouraged me to begin "peeling away the layers."

This book was inspired by author Jane Goad Trechsel who conceived of the "Morning Cup" series. Her vision, counsel, and expertise were invaluable as my thoughts turned into words on paper.

Thank you to the influential therapists, movement educators, and body workers who have supported me professionally and shared their knowledge through hands-on experience and insight, particularly Garvice Nicholson, P.T., O.C.S., and Carrie Hall, P.T., M.H.S.

My appreciation to Birmingham, Alabama's Pilates community for taking me into their hearts and homes.

A heartfelt thank you to the students who "play" with me every day. You entrust your bodies to my care and teach me how to "see" the body before me.

I dedicate this book to my nephew, Curtis, in honor of his talent, courage, and heart.

Contents

Balance Your Body with Pilates 6

Getting Started 9
    Some of the Benefits of Pilates 10
    A Little About the Routine 11

Preparing Your Body 13
    Posture.. 13
    Breathing 16

The Routine 19

Bringing It All Together 70

If You'd Like to Learn More 74

About the Author 78

The Routine at a Glance 79

References 80

Balance Your Body with Pilates

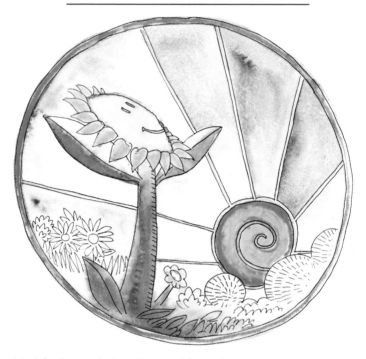

My life changed when I turned forty. I woke up one morning and knew I was going to become a physical therapist. It was a deep knowing that I never questioned in spite of the odds against me. I think there were ten applicants for every four positions in physical therapy programs across the country then, but I was undaunted. I took it one day at a time and it happened — six years later I graduated with a master's degree in physical therapy.

I became a Pilates instructor in much the same way, but this time the journey was a gift to myself. It took almost as long to complete (I'm fifty now), and it challenged me as deeply and profoundly as anything I've ever undertaken.

I discovered Pilates after a knee injury. I found that my favorite activities were painful and no longer felt good or safe. I'd always loved movement and had spent the better part of twenty years exploring different ways of moving to find an approach that met my desire for a single complete exercise discipline. I'd already done everything imaginable, including yoga, tai chi, kung fu, ballet, and dance aerobics, as well as swimming, jogging, biking, and hiking. I liked elements of each of these, but none of them seemed to meet my particular needs for one united discipline.

Then someone recommended Pilates. So I found a mat class at a local ballet studio and started practicing.

What set Pilates apart from the other exercise or movement classes I'd taken was the way the teacher taught…the words she used, the visual images she created, the personal attention she gave me through her voice or touch. She took me on a journey into my body that was incredibly enlivening. I left each class feeling renewed and rejuvenated. Best of all, my knee didn't hurt!

Pilates changed my beliefs about exercise. Before Pilates, I held a belief that I had to exhaust myself in an aerobics class to be fit, but Pilates convinced me that effective exercise didn't have to be repetitive or exhausting. I continued my cardiovascular exercise routine, but I no longer felt the need to spend hours in the gym. I started finding more time for other activities and began to look forward to daily walks as a time to reflect and to enjoy the world around me. Over time, Pilates changed my body in ways that years of jogging and the gym never achieved.

I'm only beginning to understand the implications of poor posture and movement dysfunction in my own body. It wasn't until I began participating in a regular Pilates class that my body began to change in ways that amazed even me. Postural changes inspired a new self-confidence, and I began to feel at home in my body for the first time in my adult life. As I learned more about how the body and mind are connected, I began to understand how my slumped posture was an expression of a depressed inner life (I'd suffered with depression for years).

I now have the privilege of observing students as they notice changes happening in their own bodies. Their excitement and enthusiasm as they discover a new sensation or make a new connection has helped me appreciate that movement, no matter how small or insignificant, is a wonderful way to start experiencing manageable bits of change in many areas of life. And as change is embraced, freedom is not far behind.

This book comes out of my own teaching experience and is a distillation of techniques that have worked for me in my dual role as Pilates instructor and physical therapist. The routine is a blend of Pilates-based movement and therapeutic exercise approaches I use every day in classes with people of all ages and fitness levels. I hope the routine will help you enjoy a new relationship with your body (and mind) and that you will begin to discover its many unique qualities and wonderful abilities.

Marsha K. Dorman
Birmingham, Alabama
Spring 2004

Getting Started

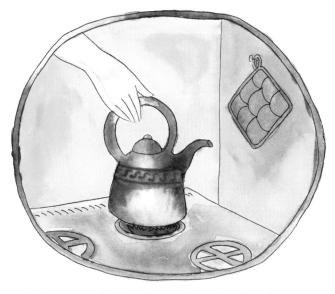

This book is intended for those of you who have been discouraged by traditional exercise classes or who simply don't have the time or opportunity to attend a class. You don't need special clothing and won't have to buy special equipment or get down on the floor. All you'll need is a chair, some wall space, and fifteen minutes in the morning or evening.

The routine is appropriate for almost anyone of any age or fitness level, even if you've been sedentary or restricted for some time, are recuperating from injury or surgery, or are fit and simply ready for something new and different. It provides a balanced and gentle movement approach to the upper and lower body that will improve range of motion and strength at most major joints as you activate your abdominal core to support better postural alignment.

Some of the Benefits of Pilates

- Better posture, alignment, and balance

- Increased flexibility and freedom of motion

- Strength and balance of the deep muscles that support the back, abdomen, pelvis, hips, and shoulders

- Relief from chronic pain conditions, including postural imbalance, repetitive use, and sports-related injuries

- Reduction in mental and physical stress

If you've been sedentary or restricted, or are dealing with stress, pain, depression, or anxiety, you will feel better, sleep better, and move better as you learn to blend breath and movement. You will learn new postural habits that, if practiced regularly, will help reduce chronic pain conditions resulting from poor alignment. If you feel unsteady or unstable on your feet, you will learn safe exercise progressions that will help you improve your balance skills.

If you are already active and fit, you will learn how to isolate and initiate movement from the deep muscular core for enhanced performance and how to use your breath to improve muscle function and movement sequencing. You will be introduced to the use of imagery to improve alignment and muscle recruitment.

> *"Self-confidence, poise, consciousness of possessing the power to accomplish our desires, with renewed lively interest in life are the natural results of the practice of (Pilates) Contrology."*
>
> Joseph H. Pilates

A Little About the Routine

✳ *Discover small movements.* Early in the routine, you will do small movements while you are learning to locate and control the small, deep "core" muscles that surround and stabilize the joints of the spine, pelvis, hips, and shoulders. These muscles are generally underdeveloped in even the very fit. The goal of these small exercises is to learn to stabilize the spine, pelvis, and shoulder girdle so you can gain full mobility and better functionality of the joints of the upper and lower limbs (hips, shoulders, knees, ankles).

✳ *Use core muscles.* These "core" muscles support standing posture, dynamic alignment, and balance. By working from muscles closer to the center or "core" of your body, the standing exercises in this routine will help make most movements safer and more efficient. This includes functional movement like walking, sitting down, reaching, lifting, or specialized sports and conditioning activities such as golf, tennis, or aerobics. By focusing on the essentials and working from the inside out, you will find your activities take on a new dimension.

> *"Developing minor muscles naturally helps to strengthen major muscles. As small bricks are employed to build large buildings, so will the development of small muscles help develop large muscles. When all your muscles are properly developed you will, as a matter of course, perform your work with minimum effort and maximum pleasure."*
>
> Joseph H. Pilates

✳ *Work on a smooth flow.* The exercises are sequenced to transition smoothly from one to the next, providing you with a continuous movement experience that strengthens and lengthens the body uniformly. If you haven't exercised in a while and the breathing causes you to feel light-headed, or if an exercise causes pain, stop and rest.

As your postural and balance skills improve, you may find that you don't have to stand next to the wall or hold onto a chair. As you build strength and endurance, you may want to add small hand or ankle weights to increase the upper or lower body challenge.

The CD that accompanies the book is paced to provide a continuous movement experience that will help you increase body awareness and practice moving from your core. In the beginning, you may want to move at a slow, continuous pace as you learn to breathe and engage your core. As you become more familiar with the routine and are able to practice safely, you can begin increasing the dynamics of the routine by adding repetitions (no more than 5-8) and making each movement extend more deeply from your core.

We've included suggestions, tips, and hints that will help you get more out of each exercise in a special section called "Special Attention" that can be found at the end of most exercises.

Use the "Routine at a Glance" provided at the end of the book for an easy reference as you are learning the exercises. Once you are familiar with the routine, you may want to use the audio CD at the back of the book, which leads you through the routine in about fifteen minutes. Review the book after you have practiced the exercises with the CD to look for cues that may help you define a movement with more clarity or go a little deeper into an exercise. Once you know the routine, pick an exercise and linger with it…take time to play with the movement, find your own internal images, add repetitions, or switch the breath to see how it changes your experience of the exercise.

Preparing Your Body

It is important to consult with your health care provider before beginning this (or any) exercise routine, especially if you have any health concerns.

For the routine, you will need two sturdy, straight-backed chairs (preferably with no arms), two firm pillows, and a kitchen or bath towel.

Posture

Place a chair in an open area that will allow enough space to reach your arms and legs to the front and out to the sides. Sit on the chair with at least half of each thigh supported on the seat.

 Place your feet flat on the floor about six inches apart, toes pointing straight ahead. It is best to have your thighs parallel to the floor. Make sure you are able to rest your whole foot (including your heel) comfortably on the ground. If you can't reach the ground with your feet, place a phone book under your feet.

Center your knees over your ankles in line with your second toe to bring your lower legs parallel to one another (this may require a slight activation of the muscles around your hips to keep your knees from falling in toward one another or out to the side). If you have a difficult time keeping your knees in place, roll up a towel and place it in between your knees as a spacer.

Make sure your pelvis and shoulders are parallel to the wall in front of you. Imagine your hip bones are headlights and your lights are shining forward. Many people maintain a slight rotation of their rib cage or shoulders, so take a moment to look down the front of your body and line up your rib cage and shoulders with your pelvis.

Bring your pelvis upright by sitting tall on your "sitting bones." Then rock slightly forward onto the front edge of your sitting bones. This position of your pelvis (a little forward of your sitting bones) and low spine (a concave curve) is NEUTRAL SPINE when you are sitting upright, and you will start most exercises from this position. Support your low back and pelvis by placing firm pillows in the space between the back of the chair and the curve of your low back (particularly important if you experience back strain or tension or have a history of low back pain). Even if you have a healthy back, the pillows will provide useful postural feedback as you practice the exercises. Your sitting bones are the bony projections at the base of your pelvis that serve as attachments for several important muscle groups including the hamstring muscles.

Breathe in. Feel your breastbone lift gently and your ribs open out and up to the sides (imagine bucket handles lifting away from the sides of a bucket). Elongate your spine down through your tailbone and reach the crown of your head up toward the ceiling to bring your rib cage upright and on top of your pelvis. Exhale to relax your rib cage.

Roll your shoulders up and back to open the front of your chest (avoid squeezing your shoulder blades together). Let your arms relax at your sides.

Lengthen your neck by reaching the tips of your ears up to the ceiling. Imagine a string attached to the back top of your head pulling it gently upward from the base of your skull, bringing your face parallel to the wall in front of you. Feel your neck as a natural extension of your spine. Imagine your head floating freely.

Sitting correctly using your postural muscles will feel like work if you normally tend to slump or fall back into an easy chair…think of how much time you spend sitting (driving a car, eating, working at a desk, sitting at a computer, watching TV, and reading). If you normally sit using poor posture, don't underestimate the work involved in simply sitting upright on a chair for a period of time. Sitting correctly is one of the most important skills to learn and practice as you adopt better postural habits…and it may be the single most important exercise you will ever do!

Breathing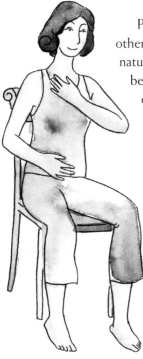

Now that you have found your correct posture, take a moment to sit quietly. Close your physical eyes and use your mind's eye to focus on your breath.

Place one hand on your chest and the other hand on your abdomen. Notice your natural breathing pattern. Do your chest and belly rise and fall gently as you inhale and exhale? Do you feel the breath move evenly into and out of your upper chest, the sides of your rib cage, and your upper and mid back? Or does your rib cage feel rigid and fixed, like a barrel? Does the breath stop at your neck, causing excess tension as your shoulders lift to get a breath in or out? Perhaps you have a habit of collapsing your chest and spine as you exhale.

Your goal is to find a breathing pattern that expands evenly throughout your rib cage…front, sides, and back…and allows you to release unwanted tension in your body, particularly the upper chest, neck, and shoulders.

For the exercises in this routine, you will breathe in through your nose and out through your mouth. Release unwanted tension as you breathe by keeping your neck long, your throat open, and your jaw relaxed.

A few things to keep in mind as you perform this series of exercises.

Keep breathing. It takes time to learn how to engage the core and to coordinate Pilates breathing with movement (kind of like rubbing your tummy and patting your head). If you find you are holding your breath or tensing up because you feel you aren't "getting it," find a relaxed breathing pattern that works for you and do what you can. Time, patience, and practice will take care of the rest.

Listen to your body. You are responsible for your body. If something hurts, review the instructions to see if you are working correctly or leave the exercise out. You can always come back to it later.

Work from the inside out. Focus more on the area of the body that is anchoring or stabilizing a movement and less on the part that is moving.

Control movement without tension. Move with ease rather than strain or tension, and stop before you reach a point of overexertion or pain.

Extra Attention

Conscious breathing is one way to begin making subtle postural changes. As you learn to breathe fully, you will begin to wake up the diaphragm and the muscles that surround your rib cage, transforming it from a rigid cage to a flexible spring that expands and releases with each breath you take.

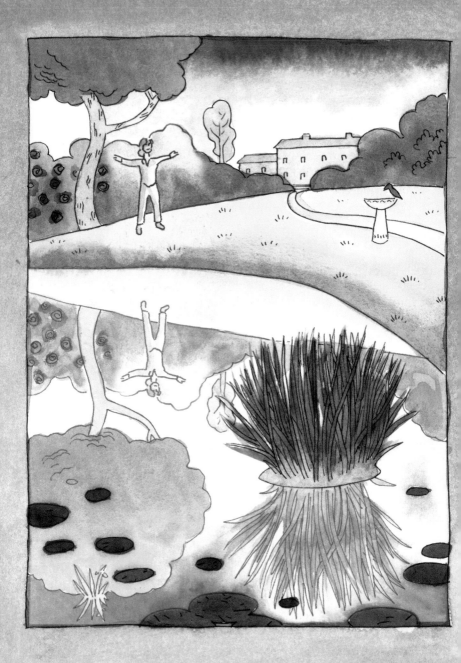

The Routine

The "core" will make you strong

The "core" fundamentals applied to the exercises in the "Morning Cup" are the underpinning of a good Pilates practice, and can be applied to any regular exercise routine. Core support refers to optimal tone in the deep, centrally located muscles that support the trunk. Core support is important because it stabilizes and controls the trunk for better posture and balance.

The Pilates "core" includes the deepest abdominal layer, called the transversus abdominus, which wraps like a deep corset around the center of your body. It also includes the pelvic floor, a muscular sling that lies at the base of your pelvic opening, spanning the area between your tail bone, sitting bones, and pubic bones. Both sets of muscles draw in to support and protect your spine. They also team up with the respiratory diaphragm to facilitate proper breathing. Clinical evidence has shown that regular participation in a Pilates class can help relieve symptoms associated with pelvic floor weakness, including incontinence and chronic low back pain.

All the poses in this routine work toward strengthening your core, as well as your other muscle groups. *Lateral Breathing, The Scoop,* and the *Pelvic Floor Lift* teach you techniques to specifically isolate and activate the important "core" stabilizing muscles.

As you integrate these exercises into your daily routine, remember to bring more awareness to how you are using your body during your regular day. Maintain an upright posture by breathing fully, and support a neutral spine by keeping your core active. As you begin to incorporate these basics into your daily activities, you will notice a difference in how you sit, stand, and move, and you will feel and look better.

Warm-up

The warm up addresses most major joints of the upper and lower body in a systematic way. It is done sitting and is great on its own if you are short of time, or want to experience your breath or develop a new awareness and appreciation of your body and how it moves. Remember to keep your pelvis neutral by sitting a little forward of your sitting bones, and support your low back by scooping your low belly, engaging your pelvic floor and using a pillow for postural feedback. If you tend to carry excess tension in your neck, shoulders, or upper back, try supporting your elbows (and lower arms) on pillows for the first several exercises.

Lateral Breathing

1. Place the heels of your hands on either side of your rib cage with elbows facing out to the sides.

2. Gently pull up on your rib cage with both hands. Breathe in and feel your ribs lift out and up into your hands, like bucket handles.

3. Press hands gently into ribs as you exhale, releasing your rib cage in toward the center of your body. Repeat 3-5 times. Don't collapse your spine or allow your shoulders to pull forward.

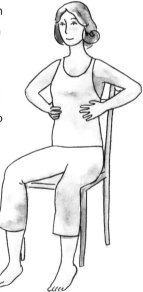

The Scoop

1. Wrap your hands around your waist just above your hip bones, laying fingers low across your belly.

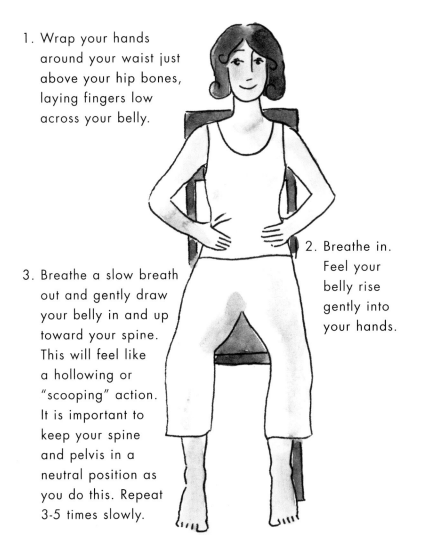

2. Breathe in. Feel your belly rise gently into your hands.

3. Breathe a slow breath out and gently draw your belly in and up toward your spine. This will feel like a hollowing or "scooping" action. It is important to keep your spine and pelvis in a neutral position as you do this. Repeat 3-5 times slowly.

Pelvic Floor Lift

(with optional shoulder blade glides)

1. Sit slightly ahead of your sitting bones. You will feel like you are sitting on soft tissue. This is your pelvic floor. Relax your arms at your sides.

2. Inhale and release your pelvic floor into the chair.

3. Exhale and gently draw your pelvic floor off the chair and up into your pelvis. Keep your pelvis neutral, don't move any bones. This is a subtle contraction of tiny muscles, not a movement of bones. Repeat 3-5 times slowly.

Optional:

For a "rub your stomach, pat your head experience" try the following to help release shoulder and neck tension. Inhale and glide your shoulder blades up as you release your pelvic floor. Exhale and release your shoulder blades as you engage your pelvic floor. Avoid actively pulling your shoulder blades down.

Shoulder Circles

1. Sit tall with your arms relaxed at your sides or supported on a pillow on your lap. Activate your core.

2. Breathe in and out as you circle your shoulders slowly in one direction.

3. Switch directions. Repeat for 2 full breaths. Smooth the circles out as you go, matching your movements to your breath. Don't hurry.

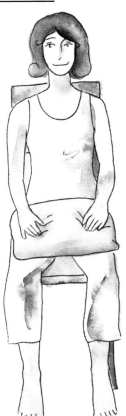

Extra Attention

Imagine hanging your shoulders from a clothesline and pulling your shoulders wider and wider along the clothesline with each repetition. Keep the circles small, about the size of a tennis ball.

Nose Circles

1. Sit tall with your arms relaxed at your sides or supported on a pillow in your lap. Activate your core.

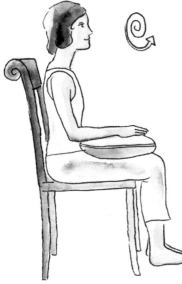

2. Place an imaginary paintbrush on your nose. Relax your jaw.

3. Breathe in and out slowly, and begin painting the wall in front of you with small, smooth nose circles that gradually spiral out.

4. Continue breathing as you reverse directions, spiraling your circles back to center. This movement is a rolling motion of the head on the neck. Repeat for one full inhale and exhale in each direction.

Extra Attention

Keep your face soft and forehead relaxed. You may want to close your eyes.

Head & Neck Rotation

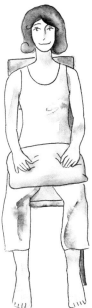

1. Sit tall with your arms relaxed at your sides or supported on a pillow in your lap. Lengthen the back of your neck. Inhale and relax your jaw.

2. Breathe out and look to the right, gently pulling your chin in the same direction.

   Breathe in, returning to center.

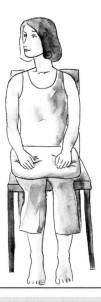

3. Breathe out and look to the left. Breathe in, returning to center. Repeat 3-5 times to each side. Keep your core active!

Extra Attention

Move your head about a vertical axis, as if you were rotating around a pole centered in your body that runs through your neck and out the top of your head.

Angel Wings

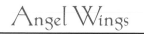

1. Relax your arms down by your sides, palms facing forward, fingers reaching, but not tense. Activate your core.

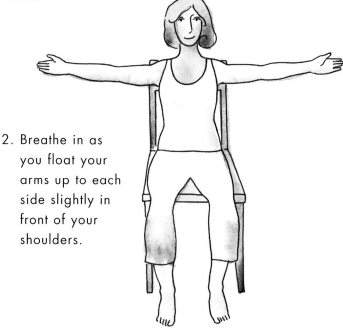

2. Breathe in as you float your arms up to each side slightly in front of your shoulders.

3. Exhale to lower your arms. Repeat 3-5 times, reaching your arms a little higher each time.

Extra Attention

Avoid actively pulling your shoulder blades down or up. Instead, feel the weight of your shoulder blades become heavier, like counterweights, as your arms rise, and become lighter as your arms lower. The shoulder blades "float" on the rib cage.

Puppet Arms

1. Raise your arms in front of your shoulders, palms facing down, elbows soft.

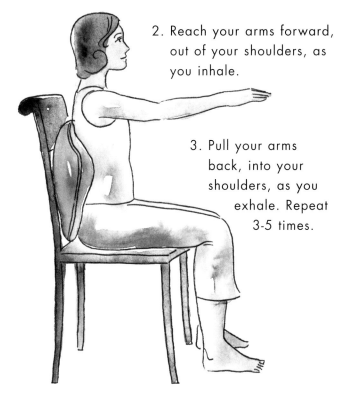

2. Reach your arms forward, out of your shoulders, as you inhale.

3. Pull your arms back, into your shoulders, as you exhale. Repeat 3-5 times.

Extra Attention

This is a gliding movement of your shoulder blades around your rib cage. See if you can feel the space between your shoulder blades broaden as you reach your arms forward and narrow as you pull your arms back.

Hug a Tree

1. Bring your arms out to each side just below shoulder level, palms facing forward.

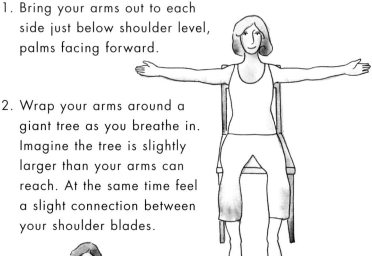

2. Wrap your arms around a giant tree as you breathe in. Imagine the tree is slightly larger than your arms can reach. At the same time feel a slight connection between your shoulder blades.

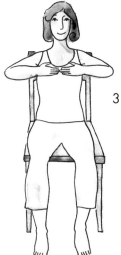

3. Breathe out as you open your arms. Keep shoulder blades wide to feel a gentle stretch through each arm. Repeat 3-5 times, keeping your neck long and shoulders relaxed. Remember to engage your core.

Extra Attention

Reach fingertips behind you by bending back at the wrist for a more intense stretch.

The Hundred

This exercise is based on the first Pilates mat exercise. It is called "The Hundred" because you pump your arms 100 times.

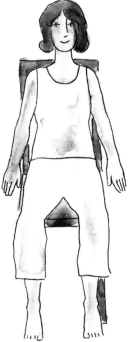

1. Lengthen arms down by your sides, palms facing back.

2. Raise arms forward slightly. Gently squeeze the backs of your upper arms and open wide across the front of your chest, pumping your arms vigorously as you inhale for 5 pumps and exhale for 5 pumps.

3. Repeat as you breathe. Start with 3-5 breaths in and out (30-50 pumps) and gradually work up to 10 breaths in and out (100 pumps).

4. Feel the core working to keep your spine steady. Stabilize your shoulder blades by drawing them forward onto your rib cage.

Extra Attention

Imagine pressing your arms through water. The vigorous pumping action is a warm-up and will get your heart pumping and blood flowing.

Inner Thigh Squeeze

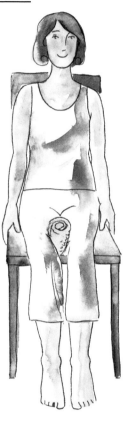

1. Bring your feet together and place a rolled-up towel between your thighs just above your knees. Breathe in.

2. On the exhale, gently engage your pelvic floor, scoop your abdominals and draw your upper inner thighs toward one another. Avoid rolling your thighs. This is a gentle isolation.

3. Inhale to release slowly. Repeat 3-5 times, keeping pelvis neutral and outer thighs relaxed. Move continuously in and out.

"Contrology (Pilates) is not a system of haphazard exercises designed to produce only bulging muscles...just to the contrary, it was conceived and tested (for over 43 years) with the idea of properly and scientifically exercising every muscle in your body in order to improve the circulation of the blood so that the bloodstream can and will carry more and better blood to feed every fibre and tissue of your body."

Joseph H. Pilates

Single Leg Stretch

1. Place a towel roll under your right thigh near the knee.

2. Inhale. Sit tall as you press your thigh into the towel roll to straighten your leg with a relaxed foot. It is important to stay upright. Avoid rounding your low back or tilting your pelvis to straighten your leg by reaching your pubic bones down and drawing your pelvic floor up.

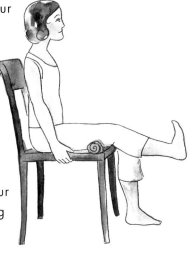

3. Exhale and flex your ankle by reaching through your heel. Inhale to point your foot. Repeat the flex/point, by bending at the ankle and keeping the toes relaxed.

4. Exhale and slowly lower your leg with a relaxed foot.

5. Switch the towel, and repeat on the left.

Knee Fold

1. Sit tall a little ahead of your sitting bones, feet 4-6 inches apart with knees centered in front of your hips. Press your hands into the sides of your chair to activate your arms and assist your core, or place your hands on your hips.

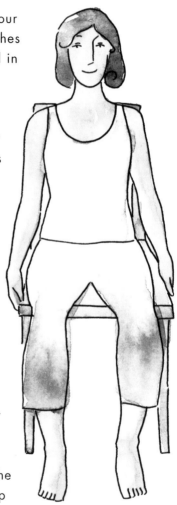

2. Breathe in.

3. On the exhale, engage your pelvic floor and press your left foot gently into the floor to float your right knee straight up. Imagine dropping your sitting bone deeper into the chair to float your knee up from a place deep inside and under the thigh. Avoid hiking your hip.

4. Inhale to lower your knee. Repeat one more time.

5. Switch sides, lifting and lowering the knee 2 times.

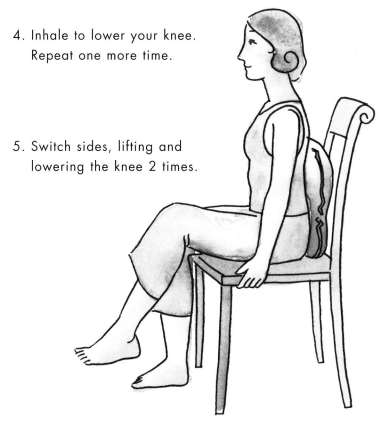

Extra Attention

It is important to maintain a neutral spine and to stabilize your pelvis as you do this exercise. Avoid rounding your low back or tilting your pelvis by reaching your pubic bones down and drawing your pelvic floor up to lift your knee. Make sure the knees don't roll in or drift past the center line of your hip.

Optional: Footwork

Footwork is an integral part of the Pilates repertoire. The ability to balance is supported by good foot and ankle alignment. Keeping the feet supple and strong provides a firm foundation for the rest of the body.

Toe Melt/Arch Support

1. Sit forward on your chair until you feel your body weight falling into your feet, knees over ankles.

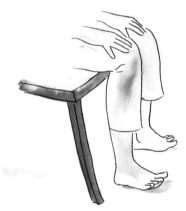

2. Lift your toes as you inhale, spreading them wide apart.

3. Melt all your toes back down into the floor as you exhale. Pull your arch up by flattening your toes and dragging them back toward your heel. Keep the big toe knuckle on the floor at all times and avoid clawing or curling your toes under. Repeat 3-5 times.

Heel Lift

1. Lift heels as you inhale, pulling them straight up the back of your calf.

2. Lower heels as you exhale. Try to keep toes melting into the floor as you lift and lower your heels. Repeat 3-5 times.

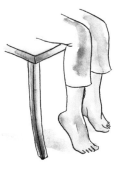

Foot Lift

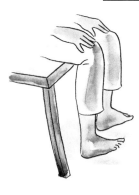

1. Lift the tops of your feet toward your shins as you inhale. Try to keep your toes relaxed and bend just at the ankle as you inhale. Hold this position.

2. Exhale to lower. Repeat 3-5 times.

Walking

1. Alternate the heel/foot lift, switching back and forth as if you were walking. Repeat 8 times.

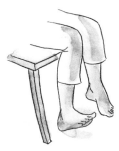

Sitting Stretches

If you have a painful low back or recent back injury, pay particular attention to your alignment as you perform these stretches. Maintain a neutral pelvis and spine by engaging your pelvic floor and scooping. Be sure to follow the directions carefully.

As you do these stretches, find a comfortable stretch sensation and hold it as you breathe slowly and continuously. Imagine your muscles lengthening and releasing with each exhale.

Spine Twist

(avoid if you've been diagnosed with osteoporosis, stenosis, a herniated disc, or spondylolysis)

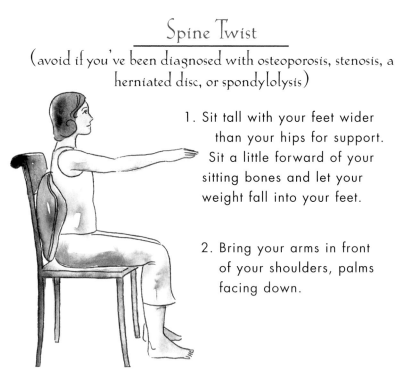

1. Sit tall with your feet wider than your hips for support. Sit a little forward of your sitting bones and let your weight fall into your feet.

2. Bring your arms in front of your shoulders, palms facing down.

3. Exhale and bend your right elbow behind you as you lift to twist your spine and rib cage to the right. Allow your head to follow. Don't force.

4. Inhale to return to center, with both arms reaching forward.

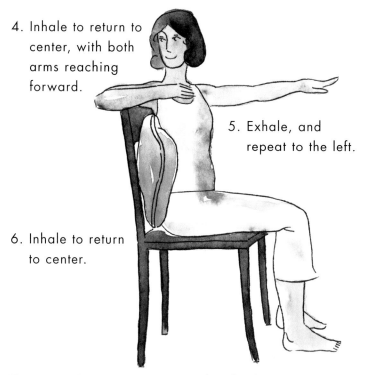

5. Exhale, and repeat to the left.

6. Inhale to return to center.

7. Repeat 2 more times on each side, keeping neck long. Imagine wringing your ribs out like a wet wash cloth as you engage your abdominal corset during each twist.

Extra Attention

It is important to face hips forward and to keep even weight on your sitting bones during these twists.

Mermaid

1. Press the heel of your right hand into your lower rib cage. Lay your left hand lightly on top of your head.

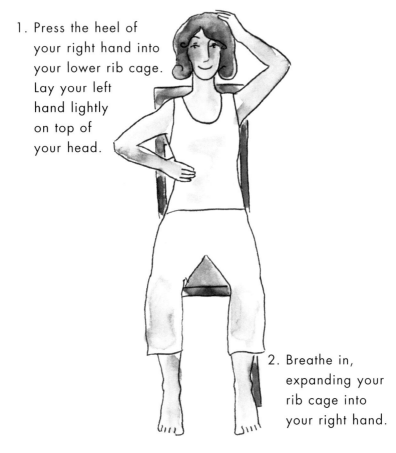

2. Breathe in, expanding your rib cage into your right hand.

Extra Attention

Open the space between each rib by gently pressing into the rib cage with the heel of one hand while you lift the other elbow to the ceiling. Stay evenly weighted on both sitting bones.

3. Breathe out and lift your rib cage up and over your right hand in a smooth side bend to the right.

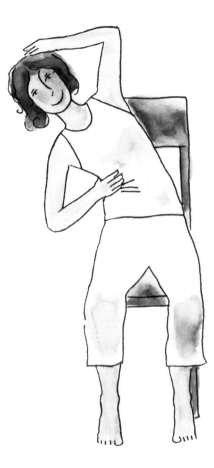

4. Reach tall as you inhale to return to center. Switch hands and repeat to the left, keeping the back of your neck long.

Ballet Stretch

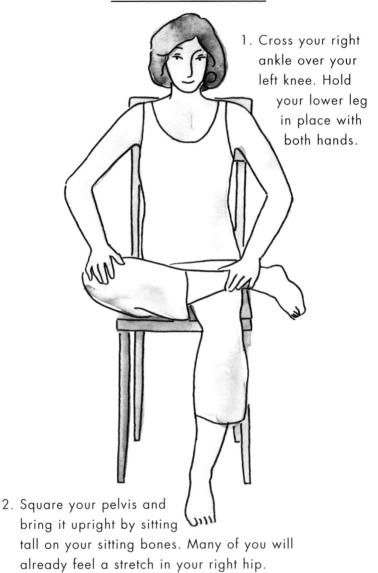

1. Cross your right ankle over your left knee. Hold your lower leg in place with both hands.

2. Square your pelvis and bring it upright by sitting tall on your sitting bones. Many of you will already feel a stretch in your right hip.

3. To increase the stretch, hinge forward at the hips by reaching your sitting bones behind you. Avoid collapsing your spine or dropping your head forward by engaging your pelvic floor and drawing your shoulder blades together slightly. Keep your head in line with your spine.

4. Hold the stretch as you breathe. Allow the tightness and tension in the back of your hip to release with your exhale for 3 breaths.

5. Repeat on the left.

Extra Attention

If this stretch is too intense or bothers your knee, place your foot on a chair in front of you with a slightly bent knee. Open your knee out to the side and bring the knee directly in front of the hip. Place a pillow or towel under the knee to support it, and hinge forward at the hips to find a stretch.

Standing Arm Series

The purpose of this series is to position your shoulder blades correctly on the rib cage as you move your arms through a full range of motion (also known as shoulder girdle stabilization). The muscles that stabilize the shoulder girdle also support the upper spine and rib cage and are critical for upright posture. These important muscles are difficult to "feel," and images are helpful as you learn to engage them. The following exercises should help bring more awareness into this area of your body.

Extra Attention

Your arms, neck, or shoulders may fatigue during this portion of the routine. Take this as a sign to rest. Build endurance over time, adding an exercise each day or lowering your arms as necessary. If these exercises cause shoulder pain, raise your arm just to the point of pain, and no further. As you build endurance, you can increase the challenge by using 1-2-pound hand or wrist weights. Sit in a chair if you want to.

Pilates V Stance

This stance is used to engage and stabilize the lower body for the Standing Arm Series. Maintain this stance as you do the next five exercises.

1. Stand with your feet parallel, about 4 inches apart.

2. Rotate your upper legs out at the hip joints to draw your heels together. Make sure you are rotating at the hips and not just at the knees or ankles. Knees and toes should follow the hips as they rotate out.

3. Draw the backs of your inner thighs up toward your sitting bones as you relax the fronts of your thighs. Keep your pelvis neutral by isolating and activating your pelvic floor and low abdominals.

Zip It Up
(Pilates V stance)

1. Bring soft fists together in front of your pelvis, arms long.

2. Breathe in by drawing your belly up and in toward your spine. Slowly pull your hands up the center of your body as if you were zipping up a tight zipper from your pubic bone to your lower ribs.

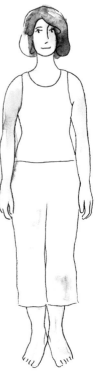

3. Exhale and press your hands back down, engaging the pelvic floor and hollowing your belly. Repeat 3-5 times.

Extra Attention

As you draw the zipper up imagine your shoulder blades floating away from your ears as your elbows rise to the sides. Avoid actively pulling your shoulder blades down.

Small Arm Circles

1. Raise your arms to the sides, slightly forward of your shoulders, palms down. Neck stays long, shoulders relaxed.

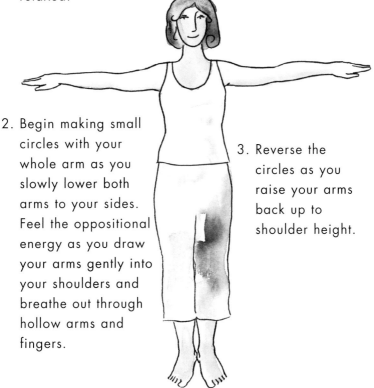

2. Begin making small circles with your whole arm as you slowly lower both arms to your sides. Feel the oppositional energy as you draw your arms gently into your shoulders and breathe out through hollow arms and fingers.

3. Reverse the circles as you raise your arms back up to shoulder height.

4. Repeat 2 times down and up. Stabilize your spine against the movement of your arms by engaging your pelvic floor and scooping your belly.

Biceps Curls Front

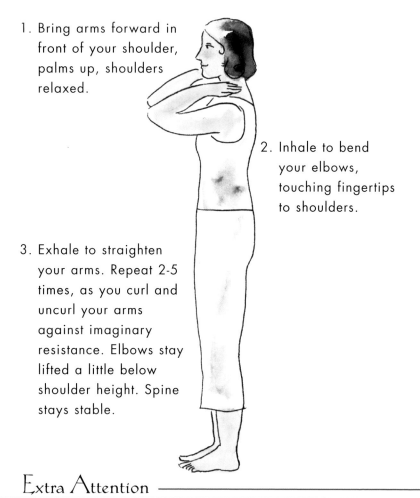

1. Bring arms forward in front of your shoulder, palms up, shoulders relaxed.

2. Inhale to bend your elbows, touching fingertips to shoulders.

3. Exhale to straighten your arms. Repeat 2-5 times, as you curl and uncurl your arms against imaginary resistance. Elbows stay lifted a little below shoulder height. Spine stays stable.

Extra Attention

Stabilize your shoulder blades by drawing your upper shoulder blades together slightly and pulling the bottom tips of your shoulder blades forward onto your rib cage until they rest under your armpits.

Biceps Curls Side

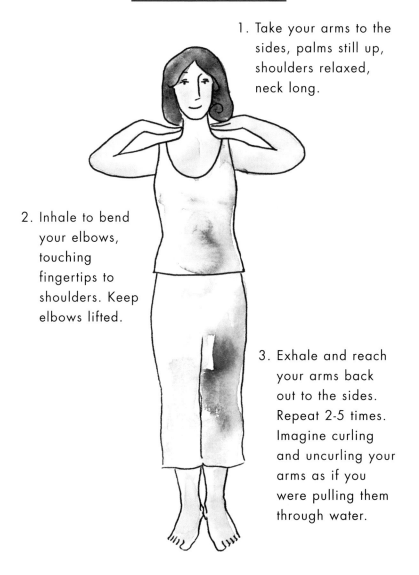

1. Take your arms to the sides, palms still up, shoulders relaxed, neck long.

2. Inhale to bend your elbows, touching fingertips to shoulders. Keep elbows lifted.

3. Exhale and reach your arms back out to the sides. Repeat 2-5 times. Imagine curling and uncurling your arms as if you were pulling them through water.

Shave Side of Head

1. Place hands next to shoulders, palms facing in. Hug elbows into sides.

2. Breathe out, straightening one arm up along your ear and the other down to your side. Keep elbows in line with shoulders as if narrow walls were pressing in on each side.

3. Breathe in, bringing elbows back to sides and hands to shoulders. Exhale to alternate arms. Repeat 3 times, keeping spine stable and core engaged.

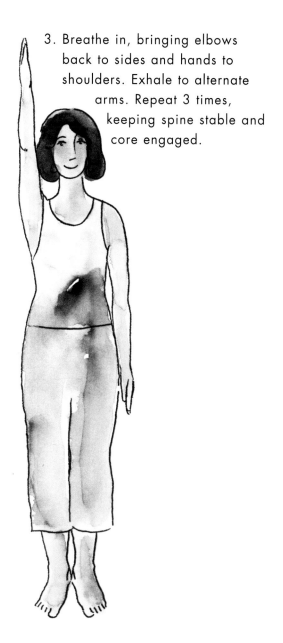

Standing Leg Series

This series focuses on balance and postural control. You will be asked to maintain a neutral upright spine and support it with your core as you move from your hips, knees, and ankles.

Bend & Stretch

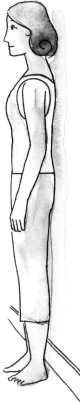

1. Stand upright against a wall with feet comfortably close to the wall. Support your mid back and pelvis on the wall by engaging your pelvic floor and drawing your belly in and up toward your spine. Keep your pelvis neutral and feel the curve of your low back and the space it makes with relationship to the wall.

2. Imagine your body is a supported plank from heels to head.

3. Inhale to sway your body slightly forward. Keep your heels on the floor and feel how your weight falls forward into the balls of your feet.

4. Exhale and bend knees over toes until you feel a slight stretch in your ankles.

5. Inhale to sway back to the wall. Your pelvis and mid back should touch the wall at the same time.

6. Exhale to slide up the wall by drawing your belly to your spine (avoid locking your knees). Repeat 1-5 times.

Lift & Lower

1. Stand upright, facing a wall. You can touch the wall with your fingers for balance.

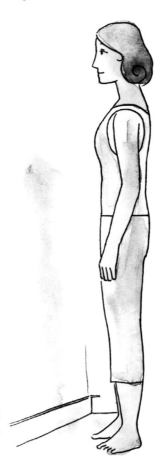

2. Feel the support of your whole foot on the floor.

3. Inhale, and draw your inner thighs up into your pelvic floor as you pull your heels straight up the backs of your calves.

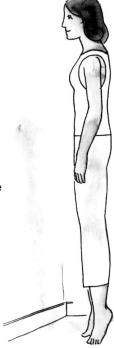

4. Exhale and continue to engage your pelvic core as you lower your heels. Feel your weight spread evenly across the ball of your foot and your toes as you lift and lower your heels. Repeat 5-8 times.

Extra Attention

If you maintain correct alignment, this exercise will build strength in the muscles that support your ankles and the arches of your feet. Notice any ankle wobble, knee bending, or balance difficulties as you lift and lower your heels. If your ankle collapses out or you tend to rock onto the outside edge of your foot as you lift up, press through the big toe and lift with the outer heel to lift up. Find more stability for this exercise using the principle of opposition…imagine lengthening your spine through the crown of your head and reaching your heels down through the floor as you rise up and down.

Stork

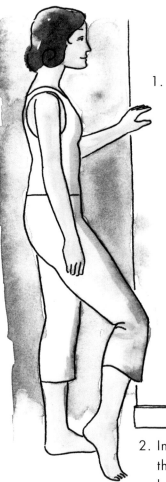

1. Stand tall with your side to the wall. Feel the strength of your hip as you bring your weight over the leg closest to the wall. Avoid falling into or pushing out into the standing hip. Instead, imagine pulling up with the inner thigh of your standing leg to align your pelvis over your hip and leg.

2. Inhale and press your arm into the wall as you pull the outer knee up to hip or waist height.

Extra Attention

Reach your pubic bones down to lift your knee up. Keep both sides of your waist long and your abdominals engaged. Don't hike your hip.

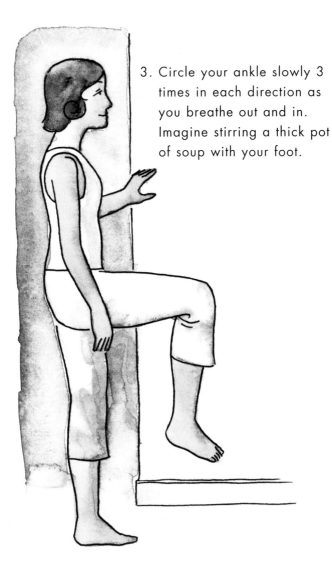

3. Circle your ankle slowly 3 times in each direction as you breathe out and in. Imagine stirring a thick pot of soup with your foot.

4. Exhale to lower the knee, and switch sides.

Clamshell

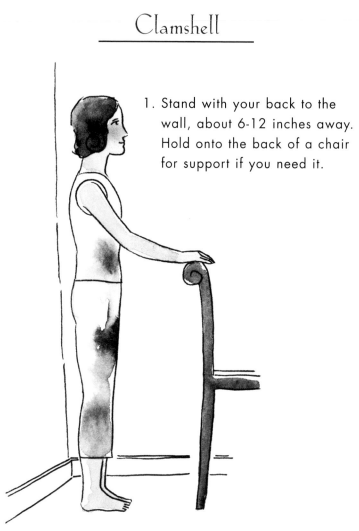

1. Stand with your back to the wall, about 6-12 inches away. Hold onto the back of a chair for support if you need it.

2. Place your foot on the wall a little below knee height with your bent knee at a 90-degree angle in front of your hip. Make sure your pelvis is level and positioned over your standing leg.

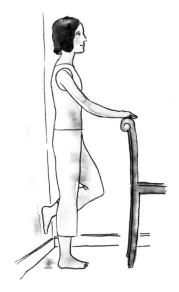

3. Inhale. Engage your core and press your foot gently into the wall, gently opening your knee to the side.

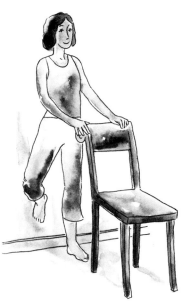

4. Exhale to close. Repeat 2 times. Switch sides.

Extra Attention

Remember to lift your knee without disturbing your pelvis. Keep your core engaged to stabilize the pelvis against the movement of the leg. Don't let the pelvis rotate.

Prancing

1. Stand tall, facing the wall with your feet directly under your hips. Touch the wall for support if you need to.

2. Inhale and lift both heels, drawing your pelvic floor and low belly in and up along your spine.

3. Exhale to lower one heel, bending the other knee.

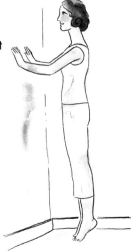

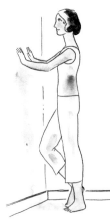

4. Inhale to lift both heels.

5. Exhale to lower the other heel. This resembles a walking motion when performed slowly. Pick up the pace as you start to warm up, breathing rhythmically, as you lift and lower 2 times with each inhale and 2 times with each exhale.

Extra Attention

This is an up-down motion. Keep your pelvis level and avoid dropping your hip or shifting side to side as you lift and lower. Imagine your pelvis is pulled up and lowered down by suspenders that pull your inner thighs up into your pelvic floor.

Balance

As you become familiar with the standing leg series, you can improve your balance by adding the following modifications:

🌿 Move a few inches away from the wall and hold onto a chair or table with two hands (then one hand). The back of the chair or table should be high enough that you can support your weight through a slightly bent elbow without having to lean forward.

🌿 Release your hand-hold and support yourself by touching the wall or chair with just one or two fingertips.

🌿 Try the exercises without holding on at all (have the wall or a chair nearby in case you lose your balance).

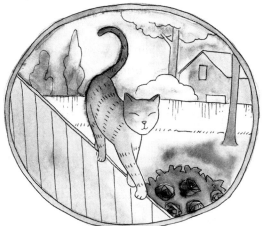

The Wall

The following exercises will help you achieve a more upright posture and help restore the natural curves of your spine if practiced regularly. This part of the routine is done against a wall for postural feedback and support. The wall will serve as a guide as you learn to engage the muscles that support upright posture, and you will use your abdominal muscles to support your spine as you move into gentle spinal flexion and extension.

Check your posture

Stand tall with your back against a wall, and your feet about 3-6 inches away from the wall. Place one hand on the wall behind your neck and the other hand on the wall behind the small of your back. Check the space between each hand and your neck and low back. If there is more than 1-2 inches of space, you may need to adjust your sitting and standing posture.

Spinal Imprinting

1. Lean tall against a wall with feet about 3-6 inches away, knees soft. Legs are parallel or in a Pilates V.

2. Inhale to expand your rib cage. Place your shoulders and head as close to the wall as possible without forcing them back to the wall. Avoid tilting your chin up to reach your head back to the wall or pressing your chin down to flatten your neck...keep your head and neck upright.

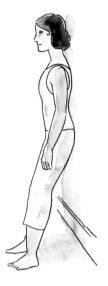

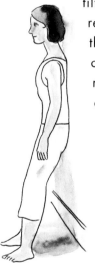

3. Exhale and draw your belly deep to your spine, gently pulling the small of your back toward the wall. This is a hollowing action of your belly and a small posterior tilt of the pelvis. Don't force your low back into the wall. Repeat slowly 3-5 times.

Extra Attention

This is a lengthening action of the small of your back accomplished by drawing your abdominal muscles up and in toward your spine. If your low back doesn't release easily, you may want to walk your feet out a few more inches and/or bend your knees slightly. Your low back will lengthen and release gradually over time.

Stick 'Em Up

1. Lean tall against a wall with feet about 3-6 inches away from the wall. Legs are parallel or in a Pilates V.

2. Exhale and draw your belly up and in toward your spine. Tilt your pelvis slightly to bring the small of your back closer to the wall. Lift your arms in the shape of a W, pressing thumbs against the wall with elbows forward of hands. Avoid shrugging your shoulders.

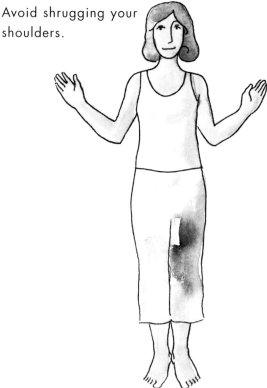

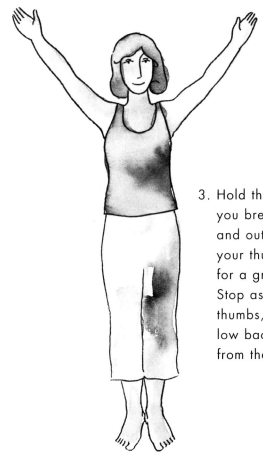

3. Hold this position as you breathe slowly in and out 3 times. Reach your thumbs up the wall for a greater challenge. Stop as soon as your thumbs, mid back, or low back pull away from the wall.

Extra Attention

Don't force your low back, arms, or head to the wall. Instead get your low back as close to the wall as you can and imagine opening across the front of your chest and shoulders. This exercise targets the postural muscles of the upper back and, if practiced daily, will help prevent a forward position of the shoulders and rounding of the upper back (called kyphosis).

Roll Down

This exercise bends your spine forward and brings your head lower than your heart. Check with your health care provider if you have glaucoma, high blood pressure, or a heart condition. Avoid forward bends if you've been diagnosed with spinal osteoporosis or a herniated disc.

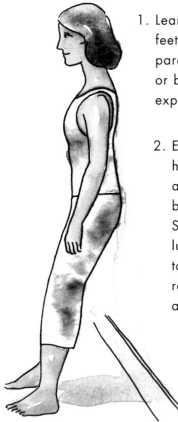

1. Lean tall against a wall with your feet 6-12 inches away. Legs are parallel or in a Pilates V. Soften or bend your knees. Inhale to expand your rib cage.

2. Exhale and begin rolling your head and spine down the wall as if you were draping your body over a large beach ball. Squeeze all the air out of your lungs and draw your ribs in toward your spine as you release your head, neck, and arms toward the floor.

3. Inhale, expanding your breath into your rib cage and back.

4. Exhale to roll back up by engaging your pelvic floor and laying each vertebra on the wall one at a time.

5. Inhale and continue rolling through your spine until your head is upright. Keep your pelvis neutral.

6. Exhale to finish. Repeat again slowly. Don't force your spine to the wall at any time...allow it to open and lengthen gradually over time.

> "Rolling and unrolling movements tend to gradually but surely restore the spine to its normal at-birth position with its correspondingly increased flexibility. At the same time you are completely emptying and refilling your lungs to their full capacity."
>
> Joseph H. Pilates

Extra Attention

A stiff, rigid, asymmetrical or unsupported spine has less ability to transmit forces effectively, causing muscular pain or joint dysfunction. This exercise improves spinal flexibility and decompresses the spine as you move your spine segmentally (one vertebra at a time) using your abdominal muscles for support. As you learn to articulate your spine using your abdominal core and the small muscles of your back, it will begin to function more like a flexible spring than an inflexible rod. Rediscovering the natural, neutral curves of your spine and developing the muscles that support these curves is a primary intent of Pilates.

Swimming

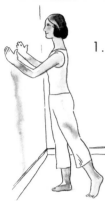

1. Stand upright facing a wall with the little finger side of your hands on the wall a little below shoulder height, elbows bent.

2. Step one foot behind you, knee relaxed, heel lifted.

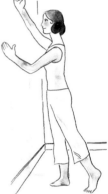

3. Inhale. Reach your heel toward the floor to straighten your leg (avoid locking your knee). Press the opposite hand up the wall by reaching through the little finger.

4. Exhale to release your arm and leg to the relaxed and bent positions. Reach and release your arm and opposite leg 2 more times. Switch sides, and do 3 times.

Extra Attention

Avoid arching your back to reach your leg. Instead, support your spine by drawing your abdominals in and up. Tip your tailbone down slightly, and reach your leg from your hip. Avoid hiking your shoulder blade to reach your arm. Instead, allow your shoulder blade to float on your rib cage as you reach through your little finger. Pull the bottom tip of your shoulder blade forward as you reach your arm higher.

Wall Push-ups

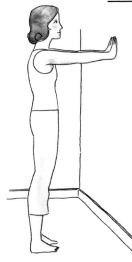

1. Stand facing a wall. Place your hands on the wall shoulder height, fingers facing up, elbows down.

2. Walk your feet away from the wall until your weight falls comfortably through your arms into the wall. Soften your elbows.

3. Imagine turning your body into a plank from your heels to your head by drawing your ribs and belly in and up toward your spine.

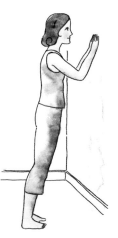

4. Inhale as you bend your elbows toward the wall, keeping shoulder blades wide and elbows narrows.

5. Exhale to press away from the wall by straightening (not locking) your arms. Repeat 4-5 times.

Extra Attention

Don't sink between your shoulder blades or arch your back as you bend your elbows. Instead, draw your belly away from the wall and in toward your spine. Feel how your abdominals support the front of your body.

Optional: Thigh Strengthener

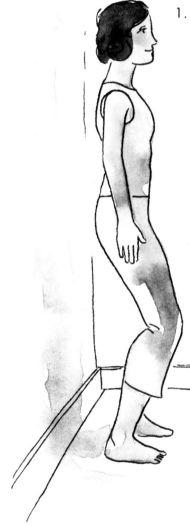

1. Stand tall with your back facing a wall and your feet hip-width apart, about 6 inches from the wall.

2. Bend your knees and draw your belly up and in toward your spine as you inhale.

3. Bend forward at the hips and reach your sitting bones behind you to touch the wall. Avoid falling backward into the wall by keeping your weight over your feet. For more challenge, bring arms to ears, keeping your back straight and your head in line with your spine.

4. Exhale and stand tall by pulling your sitting bones off the wall and pressing through your heels and drawing belly to spine. Release arms down. Don't lock out your knees.

5. Repeat, keeping weight in your heels at all times. Move a little further away from the wall as you gain strength and range of motion.

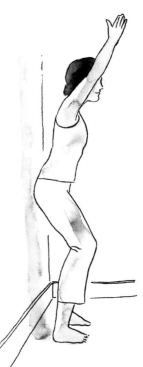

Extra Attention

This exercise is similar to sitting down and standing up. It will strengthen the muscles of your hips for all types of functional activities including lifting , going up stairs or walking uphill, picking things up off the floor, as well as pushing or pulling.

Bringing It All Together:

Improve your alignment and posture as you balance your body

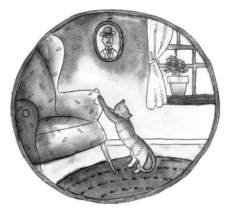

Asymmetry or handedness patterns develop in almost everyone over time. They are caused by using one side or the other to do things on a daily basis. Walking up the stairs starting with the same leg or opening doors with the same hand year after year can make you asymmetrical side to side.

Injury or poor posture can result in imbalance and asymmetry by changing the position of joints over time and restricting them, causing muscles to adapt by lengthening on one side of the joint and shortening on the other. Muscles can also become imbalanced (weak/strong, long/short) from misuse, disuse, or overuse from repetitive activities like sitting at a computer, driving, playing a sport like tennis or golf, painting, etc.

One way to deal with asymmetry or imbalance in the body is to notice how you use your body as you do daily activities. The next time you open a door or go up the stairs, notice which side you would normally use, and use the other side. If you practice a sport, find ways to strengthen the muscles on the underdeveloped side of your body. As you look at yourself in a mirror, does one shoulder droop lower than the other. Adjust your shoulders so they look more symmetrical, and try to feel which muscles you have to use to make your shoulders appear more symmetrical. Do you consistently drop into one hip while you are standing? Begin standing with equal weight on both feet. Most importantly, make an attempt to practice good posture when sitting or standing, and select several exercises in this book to do if you sit at a desk all day.

> *"Standing is also very important and should be practiced at all times until it is mastered. First, assume the correct posture, then when tired shift the weight of the body from one side to the other while resting on the "idle" side. Do not push your hips out or lock your knees. Progress forward with a slightly swaying graceful motion comparable to the effect created by a gentle breeze blowing over a field of growing wheat ready for harvest, causing it to gracefully sway in "waves" from its roots to its tips."*
>
> *Joseph H. Pilates*

Poor Posture and Back Pain

Years of slouching into your upper back, hanging your head, pushing your pelvis forward, and locking your knees can cause your spine to lose its natural curves. If your lower abdomen sags or protrudes and your typical spinal posture in standing and sitting is not neutral, you are adding abnormal stresses to the bones of the spine and making excess demands on the muscles that support the spine.

If left unchecked, postural imbalances can result in big problems over time. Poor alignment combined with muscular imbalances can place enough stress on a joint that it will begin to deform, causing cartilage destruction and painful osteoarthritis (especially true of the spine, hip, knee, and shoulder joints).

Hips and legs are the workhorses of the body, not your back. Cultures like ours that provide comfortable furniture to sit and recline on reduce the need for internal postural support. Hip joints get stiff and weak because they are no longer required for squatting or climbing or getting up off the floor. Lack of hip mobility and strength sends strain to other parts of the body that are required to compensate for the inflexibility and weakness of the hips, including the spine, knees, and shoulders. Cultures that encourage sitting or crouching on the floor, and vigorous climbing and walking tend to foster good alignment and strong hips and legs.

Tips for Lifting, Carrying, Pulling, Pushing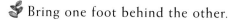

Learn to bend at the hips and knees rather than the waist to pick things up off the floor or to do daily tasks like vacuuming and laundry. Rounded shoulders are a clue that you are bending at the wrong place. Maintain a "neutral spine," support it with your pelvic core, and use the power of your legs and hips to do your daily tasks.

Tips for Getting Out of a Chair

It is important to feel the weight of your upper body in your feet when you stand up and sit down. Bringing the weight of your body forward into your feet allows you to use the strength of your legs and hips rather than your back to perform these common actions.

- Bring one foot behind the other.

- Sit upright a little forward of your sitting bones. Bend forward at the hips until your feel your weight fall forward into your toes and the fronts of your feet. Keep your back straight and head in line with spine.

(Place your hands on your thighs or the arms of a chair if you need more support.)

 Stand by pulling your belly in toward your spine and pressing both feet firmly into the floor.

Tips for Standing

Take a moment to notice your typical standing posture. Do you tend to slouch, lock your knees, stand with your weight on one leg, or push your hips forward when you stand. Weight-bearing joints such as the knees and hips cannot serve as shock absorbers if you lock them or "hang" on them and forces will be transmitted improperly through the joints, weakening them and making them vulnerable to injury. Instead, stand upright and balance the weight of your upper body directly over your hips, knees, and ankles. Feel the weight of your body fall equally into both feet. Soften your knees rather than locking them. Avoid continuous use of shoes with higher heels...even a one-inch difference changes the normal curves of the spine and places abnormal stresses on the hips, knees, and feet.

If You'd Like to Learn More

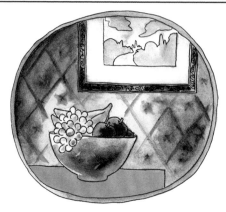

A *Morning Cup of Pilates* provides many of the basics you will find in an introductory Pilates class, but it's not meant to substitute for a traditional class or private session with an instructor. As you dive into the Morning Cup and begin to experience some of the benefits of a daily practice, I hope you will be curious to learn more. The following section may answer some of the questions you have about Pilates and help you understand more about how Pilates might benefit you.

Pilates, like other mind-body techniques, uses breath and movement patterns to peel away the layers of physical stress, tension, and holding patterns that most of us develop over time. As this layer of outer tension releases, you will begin to retrain muscles and build in new patterns of muscle usage by repeating specific whole-body movement patterns. This sequenced movement will begin to imprint new ways of moving deep into your muscle, mind, and memory. Pilates helps repattern muscle imbalances and free restriction by working muscle groups simultaneously and uniformly using the breath and proper alignment.

> *"Through contrology (Pilates) you purposely acquire complete control of your body and then through proper repetition of its exercises you gradually and progressively acquire that natural rhythm and coordination associated with all your subconscious activities...."*
>
> Joseph H. Pilates

Use the Breath to Unite Body and Mind

Using the breath consciously is a fundamental skill common to mind-body disciplines like Pilates, yoga, and tai chi. Take a moment to become aware of your breath. Can you describe its qualities (shallow, deep, erratic, regular, effortful, relaxed, light, heavy)? As you attend to it, does it change or takes on different qualities? Often what starts as effortful, shallow, or erratic breathing becomes easier, deeper, and more relaxed as you pay attention to it.

That's because breath is one of the few automatic functions that we can bring under conscious control. This gives us the ability to consciously alter our breathing pattern to affect our feelings or thoughts, to alter physiological processes such as heart rate or blood pressure, and to balance overall muscle tone. Perhaps you live a life that has many demands, and you periodically suffer from stress or anxiety that leads to nagging shoulder or neck tension.

As you begin a regular breathing practice as part of your Pilates practice, you may find that conscious breathing helps you feel calmer and relaxes your body, helping to decrease muscle tone in areas that normally tense up and get tight. On the other hand if you are just getting back to exercise and feel that you have no muscle tone, or you feel a lack of motivation and energy, you will be amazed to find how you can use conscious breathing to activate and energize the body, increasing muscle tone and supporting more efficient postural alignment.

Detoxify and Free the Body and Breath

Joseph Pilates intended his method to detoxify and stimulate the organs and tissues of the body, using dynamic movement and rolling and unrolling movements of the spine to open the body and increase circulation to every cell of the body. He called this effect "the internal shower."

Years of poor posture can result in a compressed and inflexible rib cage that limits movement of the diaphragm. The body must expend more energy just to breath. Years of sedentary living as well as the effects of injury or surgery can compress and decrease movement at joints, compress organs and the tissues that surround joints, limiting circulation into and out of tissues. Nutrients can't efficiently get into tissues and organs, and toxic substances can't escape. Organs respond by shutting down, and tissues respond by getting stiff and painful. Moving joints and muscles through coordinated movement patterns can help open and support the systems of the body, kind of like a self-massage.

> *"Contrology is not a system of haphazard exercises designed to produce only bulging muscles...just to the contrary, it was conceived and tested (for over 43 years) with the idea of properly and scientifically exercising every muscle in your body in order to improve the circulation of the blood so that the bloodstream can and will carry more and better blood to feed every fibre and tissue of your body."*
>
> *Joseph H. Pilates*

As your body opens and circulation improves to all tissues of the body, you will be able to activate and gain more control over the smaller muscles that support joints and control movement. As you gain deep muscular control closer to the center of your body, you will be able to coordinate complex movement patterns with greater precision and dynamics. This will make it possible to safely learn more challenging exercises and build speed and dynamics into your workout.

Controlling movement from a strong center rather than moving unconsciously or haphazardly sets Pilates apart from other forms of exercise, resulting in economy of movement in all your daily activities and fewer injuries.

> *"The complete exhalation and inhalation of air stimulates all muscles into greater activity."*
>
> *Joseph H. Pilates*

Increase energy and efficiency by "working from the inside out" Sometimes muscles farther from the center will substitute for muscles closer to the center, setting you up for pain or injury and expending more energy. Take a second to run through your inner checklist. Are you hiking your shoulders up around your ears to lift your arm? Are you tensing your neck to breathe? Are you gripping your back to lift your leg?

Increasing tone in the muscular core supports joints farther away from the core (spine, shoulders, knees, and hips). If you have chronic shoulder tension, you may find that increasing tone in your core stabilizing muscles can help release your shoulder tension. If you have chronic back pain, you may find that increasing tone in your core will help support your spine. Over time, as you learn to work from your center, you may be able to find a sense of ease in back, neck, and shoulder muscles. As these overworking muscles relax and release, you may find that you have more energy for other activities.

About the Author

Marsha Dorman is a physical therapist. She is also a registered instructor and member of the Pilates Method Alliance, qualified to teach the full Pilates repertoire on the mat and apparatus.

Marsha experienced the benefits of Pilates as a tool for wellness and rehabilitation while recovering from a knee injury that kept her from participating in her regular fitness activities.

In 1998, she completed a series of courses offered by Polestar Education, a Pilates program for rehabilitation professionals. She continued her Pilates education with Rachel Taylor Segel and Amy Taylor Alpers (authors of *The Everything Pilates Book*) at the Pilates Center in Boulder, Colorado, and was certified as a Pilates instructor in 2002.

Marsha lived and taught Pilates mat classes and private sessions in Birmingham, Alabama, for four years, where she was instrumental in developing the Pilates-based movement and post-rehabilitation program at St. Vincent's Hospital Fitness and Wellness Center.

Marsha now lives in Seattle, Washington, where she continues to seek safe and effective ways to integrate Pilates-inspired movement education into the rehabilitation environment.

The Routine at a Glance

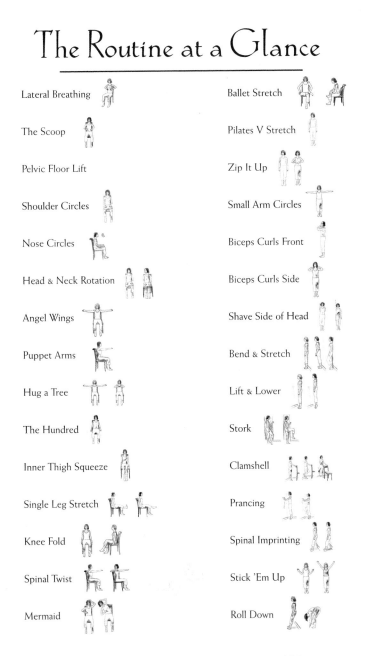

Lateral Breathing

The Scoop

Pelvic Floor Lift

Shoulder Circles

Nose Circles

Head & Neck Rotation

Angel Wings

Puppet Arms

Hug a Tree

The Hundred

Inner Thigh Squeeze

Single Leg Stretch

Knee Fold

Spinal Twist

Mermaid

Ballet Stretch

Pilates V Stretch

Zip It Up

Small Arm Circles

Biceps Curls Front

Biceps Curls Side

Shave Side of Head

Bend & Stretch

Lift & Lower

Stork

Clamshell

Prancing

Spinal Imprinting

Stick 'Em Up

Roll Down

References

Books

Classic Pilates:

Amy Taylor Alpers & Rachel Taylor Segel. *The Everything Pilates Book*. Adams Media Corporation, 2002.

Kellina Stewart. *Pilates for Beginners*. Carroll & Brown Publishers, 2001.

Brooke Silar. *The Pilates Body*. Broadway Books: a division of Random House, 2000.

Sean Gallagher & Romana Kryzanowska. *The Pilates Method of Conditioning*. BainBridgeBooks, 1999.

Modern Pilates:

Penelope Latey. *Modern Pilates*. Allen & Unwin, 2001.

Sally Searle & Cathy Meeus. *Secrets of Pilates*. DK Publishing, Inc., 2001.

Anna Selby & Alan Herdman. *Pilates Body Conditioning*. Barron's Educational Series, Inc., 1999.

Pilates for Special Populations:

Karena Thek Lineback. *OsteoPilates*. New Page Books: a division of The Career Press, Inc., 2003.

Sherri R. Betz, P.T. *The Osteoporosis Exercise Book*. Osteo Physical Therapy, 1999.

Websites (Instructors, Training, Equipment)

Pilates Method Alliance (instructors, training programs)
www.pilatesmethodalliance.org

The Pilates Center - Boulder (instructors, training program)
www.thepilatescenter.com

Polestar Education (videos, instructors, training programs)
www.polestareducation.com

Balanced Body (videos, books, equipment, training programs)
www.pilates.com

Stott Pilates (videos, books, equipment, instructors, training programs)
www.stottpilates.com